Power to
the Patient

Power to the Patient

Selected Health Care Issues and Policy Solutions

Edited by
Scott W. Atlas, M.D.

Contributors
Scott W. Atlas, M.D.
Daniel P. Kessler
Mark V. Pauly

HOOVER INSTITUTION PRESS
Stanford University   Stanford, California

Hoover Institution Press Publication No. 532

First printing, 2005
12 11 10 09 08 07 06 05   9 8 7 6 5 4 3 2 1

Manufactured in the United States of America

The paper used in this publication meets the minimum requirements of the American National Standard for Information Sciences—Permanence of Paper for Printed Library Materials, ANSI Z39.48–1992. ♾

Library of Congress Cataloging-in-Publication Data

Power to the patient : selected health care issues and policy solutions
   / edited by Scott W. Atlas ; contributors, Scott W. Atlas, Daniel
   P. Kessler, Mark V. Pauly.
      p. ; cm.— (Hoover Institution Press publication ; no. 532)
      Includes bibliographical references and index.
      ISBN 0-8179-4592-X (alk. paper)
      1. Medical care, Cost of—United States.   2. Medical care—United
   States—Cost control.   3. Insurance, Health—Economic aspects —United
   States.   4. Medical savings accounts—United States.   5. Medical
   policy—United States.   I. Atlas, Scott W., 1955–   .   II. Kessler,
   Daniel P.   III. Pauly, Mark V., 1941–   .   IV. Series: Hoover Institution Press
   publication ; 532.
      [DNLM: 1. Health Care Costs—United States.   2. Health Expenditures—
   United States.   3. Health Policy—United States.   4. Insurance, Health—
   economics—United States.   5. Medical Savings Accounts —United States.
   W 74 AA1 P887 2005]
   RA410.53.P685 2005
   362.1'0425'0973—dc22   2004023120
   [ISBN 0-8179-4592-X]

Contents

Contributors

SCOTT W. ATLAS is a senior fellow at the Hoover Institution and professor of radiology and chief of neuroradiology at Stanford University Medical School.

Atlas's research interests at Hoover focus on issues pertaining to public policy in health care. He is investigating the ways of increasing direct patient payments for health care so that free market effects can play out on prices. His work also includes investigations into the effect of the changing health care marketplace on technology-based innovations in medicine, with special emphasis on the effect of managed care on expensive techniques involved in emerging medical applications.

Atlas is the editor of the leading textbook in the field, the best-selling *Magnetic Resonance Imaging of the Brain and Spine*. He is also editor, associate editor, or member of the editorial boards of many scientific journals and has been a member of the boards of major scientific societies over the past decade. Atlas has written more than one hundred scientific publications in leading journals. He has lectured throughout the world on various topics, most notably on advances in brain imaging and on economic issues related to the future of such technology-based advances. He is also an adviser to industry leaders in medical technology. Atlas has received many awards and honors in recognition of his leadership in the field.

Before his appointments at the Hoover Institution and Stanford University, Atlas was on the faculty of the University of California at

San Francisco, University of Pennsylvania, and Mount Sinai Medical Center in New York City.

Atlas received a B.S. degree in biology from the University of Illinois in Urbana-Champaign and an M.D. degree from the University of Chicago School of Medicine.

DANIEL P. KESSLER is a professor at the Stanford University Graduate School of Business, a senior fellow at the Hoover Institution, and a research associate at the National Bureau of Economic Research. He has a J.D. from Stanford Law School and a Ph.D. in economics from the Massachusetts Institute of Technology. His research interests include antitrust law, law and economics, and health economics. His current research, in addition to work on using claims data to detect Medicare abuse, focuses on the effect that organizational form in health care has on the cost and quality of care.

MARK V. PAULY holds the position of Bendheim Professor in the Department of Health Care Systems at the Wharton School of the University of Pennsylvania. He received a Ph.D. in economics from the University of Virginia. He is professor of health care systems, insurance and risk management, and business and public policy at the Wharton School and professor of economics in the School of Arts and Sciences at the University of Pennsylvania. Dr. Pauly is a former commissioner on the Physician Payment Review Commission and an active member of the Institute of Medicine. One of the nation's leading health economists, Dr. Pauly has made significant contributions to the fields of medical economics and health insurance. His classic study on the economics of moral hazard was the first to point out how health insurance coverage may affect patients' use of medical services. Subsequent work, both theoretical and empirical, has explored the effect of conventional insurance coverage on preventive care, on outpatient care, and on prescription drug use in managed care. He is currently studying the effect of poor health on worker productivity. In addition, he has explored the influences that determine whether insurance coverage is available and, through several cost-effectiveness studies, the influence of medical care and health practices on health outcomes and cost. His work in health policy deals with the appropriate design for Medicare in a budget-constrained environment and the ways to reduce the number of uninsured through tax credits for public and private insurance. Dr. Pauly is co-editor-in-chief of the *International Journal of Health Care, Finance, and Economics* and associate editor of the *Journal of Risk and Uncertainty*. He has served on the Institute of Medicine panels on improving the financing of vaccines and on public accountability for health insurers under Medicare. He is an appointed member of the U.S. Department of Health and Human Services National Advisory Committee to the Agency for Healthcare Research and Quality (AHRQ).

Preface

Health care represents one of the most important domestic issues facing the American people. There is little question that most technological advances, physician training, and leadership in research and development in medical care occur in the United States. It is also widely recognized that most American physicians would do everything possible to have their medical care back home if they were to become seriously ill overseas. However, despite widely recognized leadership in many areas of medicine, the American health care system has significant problems.

Increasing costs, accompanied by dissatisfaction with the system from patients, doctors, and employers, have put reform on the agenda. Managed care during the 1990s shifted control to nonmedical bureaucrats, failed to stabilize expenditures, added more administrative complexity and cost to the system, and further distanced patients from controlling their own health care dollars. Despite the clear failure of top-down management of health care in America, much of the debate about solutions still focuses on expanding government control and on further shifting power to third-party payers. We are at a critical point in time with this issue. Indeed, there is a unique opportunity to introduce major changes to the American health care system.

This monograph stems from a recent Director's Seminar held at the Hoover Institution in Stanford, California. In that symposium, three speakers put forth their views on three key topics in health care. Professor Scott Atlas, senior fellow of the Hoover Institution and professor in the Stanford University School of Medicine, outlined fundamental reforms for the health care system, centering on empowering the patient and eliminating the third-party payer. Professor Daniel Kessler, senior fellow of the Hoover Institution and professor in the Graduate School of Business at Stanford University, discussed the effects of medical liability and the legal system on medical expenditures. Professor Mark Pauly of the Wharton School of the University of Pennsylvania discussed rising health care expenditures. These ideas are expanded in this monograph.

The purpose of this monograph is to highlight important issues in the current American health care system; the topics discussed in these articles are not intended to be all-inclusive of the numerous problems in the system. The Hoover Institution hopes that these writings will spark further debate and help generate significant reform in what most American citizens and physicians regard as one of America's most important assets.

Scott W. Atlas, M.D.
Senior Fellow, Hoover Institution

Acknowledgments

This monograph and the Director's Seminar on Health Care held at the Hoover Institution in Stanford, California, on November 10, 2003, were supported in part by generous support from Robert and Marion Oster.

Chapter One

Power to the Patient: The Right Choice to Control Health Care Costs

Scott W. Atlas, M.D.

Background

There is little question that health care was near the top of the list of domestic issues in the minds of voters in this past year's presidential election. Unfortunately, health care is one of the more complicated issues to address. Patients, doctors, and employers are dissatisfied with the current system, which they view as bloated, unnecessarily complex, restrictive, and at the same time increasingly costly. Proposed solutions to these problems run the gamut from loosely defined, consumer-driven plans to a single-payer system with broad government control. This diversity of opinion on health care often masks the widely shared goals of high-quality medical care, broad access, and affordability.

As the debates reverberate over how to cope with the rising cost of medical care, advanced medical technology—often but erroneously blamed as the fundamental driver for increasing medical care expenses—continues to progress at a remarkable rate. Opinion leaders in health care estimate that technology, more than any other factor in the year 2010, will have a dramatic effect on health care.[1] Despite dissatisfaction and frustration with the current system, patients recognize that many technology-based medical innovations have been remarkably effective.[2]

Public appreciation of the benefit from medical innovations has been accompanied by a belief that Americans are entitled to immediate and broad access to the most sophisticated health care technologies, regardless of cost. How has this unsustainable belief arisen? The third-party system of payment—the absence of direct payment from patient to doctor for most medical expenses—has shielded Americans from considerations of cost and imparted the illusion that "someone else is paying" for medical care. The forces of supply and demand have become lost amid the sea of governmental regulation and oversight in the third-party payer system. The essential step to remedy this is to change the nature of health care insurance so that *patients make direct payments to their health care providers.*

The United States has the costliest health care system in the world on a per capita basis. The growth of managed care in the 1990s, in an attempt to control rising health care costs, temporarily stabilized insurance premiums as well as national health care expenditures. However, average insurance premiums are once again rising by 10 to 15 percent a year, and health expenditures are predicted to increase by more than 16 percent of the gross domestic product (GDP) by 2007 and to double by 2012.[3] Yet rising expenditures on

---

1. "HealthCast 2010: Smaller World, Bigger Expectations," Pricewaterhouse-Coopers, November 1999.

2. D. M. Cutler and M. McClellan, "Is Technological Change in Medicine Worth It?" *Health Affairs* 11 (September/October 2001): 29.

3. K. Davis and B. Cooper, "American Health Care: Why So Costly?" June 11, 2003, Invited Testimony, Senate Appropriations Committee, Subcommittee on Labor, Health, and Human Services, Education and Related Agencies, Hearing on Health Care Access and Affordability: Cost Containment Strategies.

health care are not confined to the United States. On the contrary, Organization for Economic Cooperation and Development (OECD) data have shown that the universal trend in developed nations is for medical care costs to increase.[4] It is notable that health care markets in the rest of the world are more government-controlled than in the United States.

Thanks to advances in medical care and sanitation, pharmaceutical breakthroughs, and lifestyle changes—all contributing to better health and declining birth rates—the population is aging (see figure 1.1).[5] Since elderly patients are responsible for a large fraction of medical care costs, we seem to be headed for an unaffordable system.

Why worry about high health care costs? After all, few expenditures are more important to society. Moreover, as medical innovation continues, there may be unavoidable costs associated with their use, particularly on their first introduction. This is generally a good thing; developing more effective medical care is a major goal of modern society. In the end, more effective medical care may indeed be less costly, for example, medical instead of surgical therapy or minimally invasive treatment resulting in shorter hospital stays. Clearly, as nations become wealthier, their citizens spend more money on health care.[6] Similarly, people spend more on houses, cars, clothes, and so on, as their income increases. The argument that high and rising health care costs are bad for people needs to be considered in context. People are spending more money on cars, houses, and Internet-related technologies—this has not necessarily been a bad thing. Insofar as people get something that they value for the extra money that they spend on medical care, it *adds* to their real income.

---

4. *Health at a Glance: OECD Indicators*, 2003.

5. "World Population Prospects" (1999 revision), United Nations Population Division, Dept. of Economics and Social Affairs, New York 1999.

6. Robert J. Maxwell, *Health and Wealth: An International Study of Health Care Spending*, (Lexington, MA: Lexington Books, 1981); B. Abel-Smith, "Escalation of Healthcare Costs: How Do We Get There?" OECDHealthcare, Paris, 1996.

Figure 1.1   Share of Population Aged 65 and Older in Selected Developed Countries (2000) and Change in Share (1960–2000)

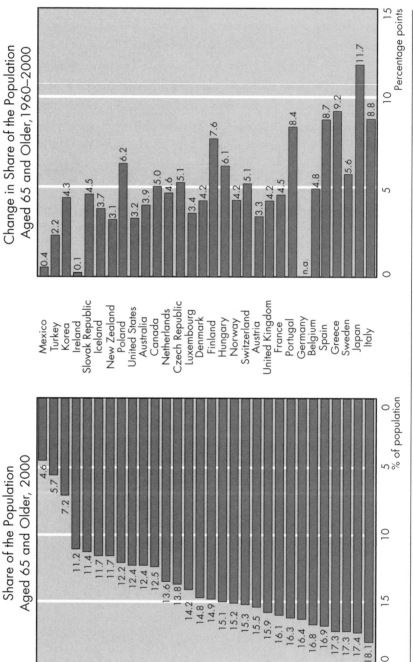

Share of the Population
Aged 65 and Older, 2000

Change in Share of the Population
Aged 65 and Older, 1960–2000

Source: Health at a Glance: OECD Indicators, 2003.

Attempts to control costs by limiting services or setting prices misalign incentives and invariably result in supply shortages—this is well documented in history, and the health care industry is no different. At the same time that the United States is leading the world into a new era in medicine with the convergence of molecular biology, medical imaging, and minimally invasive diagnosis and therapy, we have seen an alarming trend toward using technologies that are not state-of-the-art and toward reducing the availability of improved technologies with managed care penetration.[7] These top-down regulatory approaches reduce access to advanced medical technologies and will affect our high standards and expectations of the American health care system.

How Can We Empower the Patient?

The critical focus should be on putting consumers in charge of the money and letting them make cost-conscious decisions about spending health care dollars. During this past presidential primary season, six Democratic presidential candidates have outlined proposals to broaden health insurance coverage. According to a September Commonwealth Fund publication, Democratic plans have estimated costs to the federal budget ranging from $590 billion to $6 trillion over a ten-year period.[8] Senator Kerry's plan is estimated to add $895 billion in cost to the system over ten years.[9] Mr. Kerry's plan also involves shifting the cost from employers and employees to taxpayers by shifting the role of the insurer from the insurance companies to the government. Expanding third-party coverage increases bureauc-

---

7. L. Baker and S. W. Atlas, "Diffusion and Utilization of MR Scanners and Managed Care," *Journal of the American College of Radiology* 1 (2004): 478–487.

8. Sara R. Collins, Karen Davis, and Jeanne M. Lambrew, *Health Care Reform Returns to the National Agenda: The 2004 Presidential Candidates' Proposals*, Commonwealth Fund Publication, September 2003.

9. See note 8.

racy and further distances patients from paying for their own medical care. It strengthens the role of the third-party payer. This is the wrong approach. It is time to give the ownership of medical care to the patient and to expose health care to free market competition.

Out-of-pocket expenses for health care are highly important to consumers—the consideration of price is an essential part of a free market economy, and health care is no exception. A number of studies, most notably the "Rand Health Insurance Experiment" conducted from 1974 to 1982, have demonstrated that the more people have to pay for medical care without insurance reimbursement, the less they spend on total medical care. In 1960, more than 55 percent of health care costs were paid directly by the consumers of that care. Currently, third-party payers pay an unprecedented 85 percent of health care costs. This system encourages patients to neglect cost and to overspend for medical care. The separation of the patient from his medical care bills has meant less choice for the consumer: 40 percent of all employers and a full 92 percent of small employers offer only a single choice of health insurance. Yet while many nations seem to be privatizing, the American consumer is increasingly shielded from paying for medical care.[10] Trends show that in the United States, more than in any other country, consumers paid significantly less out-of-pocket in the 1990s (see figure 1.2). This trend of decreasing out-of-pocket expenditures has continued through 2002.[11]

The recently enacted Medicare Prescription Drug Improvement and Modernization Act of 2003 contains two extremely important provisions that have broadened coverage and empowered patients. The Medicare Act defines 1) high-deductible health plans (HDHP) and 2) tax-favored Health Savings Accounts (HSA) to be used in

---

10. See note 4.
11. K. Levit et al., *Health Affairs* 23 (2004): 147–159.

Figure 1.2 Out-of-Pocket Outlays for Health Care

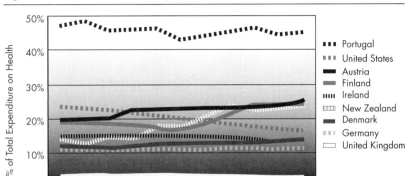

Source: OECD Health Data 1998.

conjunction with a qualified high-deductible plan. The law has established that HDHPs must have a minimum deductible of $1,000 for individuals and $2,000 for families. The main effect has been to reduce the cost of health insurance by changing the role of health insurance to provide coverage for unanticipated and significant expenditures. Health insurance should not cover the small expenses of *routine* medical care. We do not expect our homeowner's insurance to reimburse us when the light bulbs need replacing, or the kitchen sink is clogged, or the gutters and spouts need a yearly cleaning. Likewise, we should not expect health insurance to pay for routine maintenance and minor repairs. This change will accomplish several important goals. Most important, the patient will now pay directly for most medical expenses. By paying directly, the patient will have the responsibility and decision-making authority for how the money is spent. Incentives for value consciousness enter the decision process, since the illusion that "someone else" is paying is eliminated.

Raising deductibles will clearly make health insurance more affordable, for the employer as well as the individual. Lee and Tollen reported that a combination of 30 percent coinsurance with a $1,000 deductible would reduce premiums by 44 percent.[12] According to that study, savings in health insurance premiums would approach 50 percent by raising deductibles to $2,000. It is important to note that the cost of health insurance is reduced more by increasing out-of-pocket payments than by paring down insurance benefits. Employers paid $335 billion in health insurance premiums in 2001, and employer health expenditures have grown from 10 to 15 percent yearly since then. The high cost of health insurance has been the main contributor to the increasing number of uninsured because many employers have withdrawn health insurance from benefits packages. Of those workers who do not have health insurance, about 60 percent work for employers who do not offer this benefit.

High deductibles also will eliminate the bureaucracy and cost that accompany filing small claims. Administrative costs are projected to exceed $200 billion a year by 2012 and are rising faster than any other health care cost, aside from prescription drugs.[13] Small claims represent a large fraction of the estimated 25 percent of total health care dollars spent on administrative tasks.[14] Eliminating the burden of smaller claims will also markedly reduce the bureaucratic headaches of physicians, patients, and employers alike. Because the patient will pay directly for smaller claims, the patient becomes the customer. Third-party payers will be marginalized for most doctor-patient interactions. Patient and doctor satisfaction will undoubtedly improve because the physician will be caring for the customer

---

12. J. S. Lee and L. Tolen, "How Low Can You Go? The Impact of Reduced Benefits and Increased Cost Sharing," *Health Affairs Web Exclusive*, 2002: W229–241.

13. Levit et al., "Trends in U.S. Health Care Spending, 2001," *Health Affairs* (January/February 2003): 154–164; Heffler et al., "Health Spending Projections for 2002–2012," *Health Affairs*, February 7, 2003.

14. S. Woolander, T. Campbell, and D. Himmelstein, "Costs of Health Care Administration in the United States and Canada," *New England Journal of Medicine* 349 (2003): 768–775.

again, restoring the patient-doctor relationship. Satisfaction with the overall system will be improved for everyone.

Paying directly for health services will also diminish the notion of entitlement. As noted earlier, an unprecedented 85 percent of health care costs are paid by third parties—insurance companies, government, or employers. Shielding consumers (patients) from directly paying doctor bills has fostered the idea that patients are entitled to all medical care, regardless of cost. Insurance coverage with near-zero deductibles has implied that health care is "free." Beyond fostering an unsustainable attitude of entitlement, it has further encouraged elevated demand, since out-of-pocket costs have been minimized. One can see the effect on cost of direct patient payment in the 15 percent of today's health care marketplace where consumers pay directly for medical care. This 15 percent direct payment part of medical care is mainly encountered at the margins of the system, such as in vision and dental care or cosmetic surgery. Costs have not risen significantly for these because patients are careful about how they spend their own money; that is, when patients pay directly, they are quite successful in holding down cost increases.[15] A number of previous studies, most notably the Rand Health Insurance Experiment conducted from 1974 to 1982, have demonstrated that the more people have to pay for medical care without reimbursement, the less they spend on medical care. This is not a cause for hand wringing, as if patients were making "bad decisions" and foregoing essential medical care; to the contrary, it is simply an illustration of adult consumers making independent decisions that factor in cost. Why should it be any other way?

How would patients pay for their newly uncovered medical care? The Medicare Act of 2003 established a new tax-favored Health Sav-

---

15. G. Scanlan, "Increasing Consumer Choice in Health Care: Five Steps Employers Can Take Now," National Center for Policy Analysis, Brief No. 398, June 17, 2002.

ings Account, or HSA, as the second part of needed change in health insurance. This law allows people to deposit money for health care up to the lesser of the amount of the high deductible of the HDHP, or $2,600 for individuals or $5,250 for families. The person who owns the account, as well as others, including the employer, can contribute to the account. Deposits to the accounts would come from the difference in the cost of premiums for a low-deductible insurance policy and for the new one with a high deductible. Regulations are also outlined for the tax-free use of these accounts for qualified medical expenses and in special circumstances for other health insurance.

HSAs are designed to improve on previously established health care savings plans in significant ways. For instance, the laws for the new accounts eliminate many of the 1996 restrictions on medical savings accounts (MSAs) or similar tax-sheltered personal accounts. First, higher caps on contributions are allowed, so high deductibles can be covered. Indeed, the new contribution limits would cover what most patients spend on medical care during any single year (less than $2,000 according to survey data). A 1989 survey reported by health economists Jensen and Morlock found that nearly three-quarters of patients filed claims for less than $500 and nearly 90 percent filed claims for less than $2,000. This means nearly three of four patients would have more than $2,000 left in savings at the end of the year.

Second, the new HSAs are allowed to accumulate, tax-free, without being subject to "use it or lose it" rules. This distinguishes the new HSAs from employer-offered flexible spending accounts (FSAs), which are forfeited if they remain unused at the end of each year.

Third, HSAs are owned by the individual rather than the employer. Therefore, HSAs are portable, that is, neither tied to a specific employer nor even linked to current employment. Progress toward reducing the number of uninsured from more than 43 million Americans could be made, since many uninsured are those who have lost jobs, even temporarily.[16] Moreover, a large pool of savings would build during years when medical expenses are relatively low.

Other significant changes should be made to the health insurance industry. For instance, residents of a state are now restricted to the insurance companies in that state for their health insurance. There needs to be a national insurance market. It ought to be possible for an insurance company to be licensed federally and to operate in all states so that the customers in different states can have the benefit of competition and a wider range of alternatives. Deregulation of the insurance industry is essential in promoting competition to benefit consumers.

The New Era of Patient Empowerment

With this purchasing power comes new authority and responsibility, coinciding with the emerging era of self-directed health care. A recent study noted a clear trend toward independent decision making by health care consumers. It found that the percentage of consumers who said they followed their doctor's recommendations without question fell from 53 percent in 2000 to only 36 percent in 2002.[17] In contrast, the percentage of consumers who said they would ask their doctors to send them to the hospital that the patients themselves preferred now stands at 55 percent—up from 36 percent in 2000. Moreover, physicians—at 27 percent—rank only as the second most important source of information for patients, far behind the Internet, with 37 percent of consumers using the Internet to research hospitals, physicians, medical conditions, insurance plans, and other aspects of their own care.

Free market health care will create the appropriate incentives

---

16. Robert J. Mills and Shailesh Bhandari, "Health Insurance Coverage in the United States: 2002," U.S. Census Bureau, September 2003.

17. "National Trends in Health Care Consumerism: The Influential Health Care Consumer," Second Annual Report from Solucient, LLC, August 2003.

for discovering efficient ways to capitalize on the vast amount of information now on the Internet for both consumers and insurers. The asymmetry of medical information that has long been an obstacle to consumers is becoming much less important as the information becomes both widely accessible and virtually free. As access to online information about health and health insurance becomes widespread, the arguments against patient-directed health care become tenuous.

Can Consumers Make Appropriate Decisions about Health Care?

Medical test markets that require out-of-pocket purchase have clearly illustrated the effect of the free market and patient decision-making on health care. Recent examples include whole body CT screening, for which prices fell from about $1,200 to $300 over a two-year period.[18] In fact, an interesting argument can be made for the societal benefit of the affluent in these settings—that the affluent segment of society serves as the test market for expensive medical innovations not covered by health insurance.

Can consumers make appropriate decisions about health care? The answer is a resounding yes. Arguments to the contrary beg for comparisons to the automobile industry and to self-directed retirement accounts, industries where consumer decision making is now the status quo, despite lengthy discourse on information asymmetry. Moreover, patient empowerment through medical savings accounts will stimulate the demand for more consumer information about health care quality and pricing. These are highly positive changes. The American people should be trusted to make decisions about their own lives. Big brother attitudes do not resonate with indepen-

---

18. J. Illes et al., "Self-referred Whole Body Imaging: Current Status and Health Care Implications for the Consumer," *Radiology* 228 (2003): 346–351.

dent-minded consumers who demand to make their own critical decisions and choices about how and where to spend their money.

What about the Poor?

Raising deductibles and increasing out-of-pocket payments lead one to question how such a system, where patients pay directly for routine medical expenses up to what will be elevated levels of insurance deductibles, could work for people whose incomes fall short of leaving money for these expenses. Let us not make the mistake, which well-meaning but misguided "experts" continually fall into, of thinking that low-income families would not benefit from paying directly for their health care and choosing where their health care dollars go. There is no greater control than the control of the one who holds the checkbook. The poor are no different from everyone else in the benefits they would derive from lower health care costs, with perhaps one exception—people of low-income now subjected to restrictions on choice from government-based health insurance could enjoy much greater access and choice than their current system allows. So, despite special circumstances based on income, the overall goals and benefits for people regardless of income are at least as positive for low-income families, and potentially even more so.

Many politicians and policymakers espouse the refundable tax credit. These income-based tax credits are "refunded" to people with low income, even when their incomes are below the thresholds for any owed taxes. There is promising data that tax credits will make individual health plans affordable for millions of Americans, the working poor, who do not have access to health insurance through their employers.[19] Of the more than 62,000 health insurance plans sold by eHealthinsurance.com to people in more than forty states,

---

19. "The Cost and Benefits of Individual Health Insurance Plans," eHealthin surance.com, April 2004.

the average annual premium for an individual was about $150 a month and about $288 a month for a family of three. Of the plans purchased, more than three-fourths were Preferred Provider Organization (PPO) plans. Moreover, 94 percent of individual plans and 89 percent of family plans were "comprehensive," as defined to include inpatient, outpatient, and laboratory and test benefits: more than 75 percent also included prescription drug benefits.[20] Refundable tax credits should be aggressively promoted in conjunction with HDHPs and HSAs, available as of January 2004.

Unemployed individuals and families at or near the poverty level may not have the money to pay for routine health care that is uncovered because of the elevated deductibles. For the unemployed, the practical effect of refundable tax credits leaves much to be desired. Real life dictates that individuals and families need to meet monthly expenses and the often unexpected costs of their health care. Medical expenses do not wait until April 15 to occur. It seems highly unlikely that a once-per-year lump sum generated after tax filing time would prove sufficient for low-income families who otherwise have essentially no extra disposable cash on hand. Voucher systems and programs analogous to food stamps need to be explored, where coupons for medical care are available for very low- and no-income groups. Regardless of the specific system adopted, the goal should be to put the power of the payer directly into the hands of the patient.

Conclusions

The fundamental driver for increasing medical care spending is third-party payment. The increasing expenditures on bureaucracy, administration, and diagnosis and treatment do not derive from medical technologies but from the method of organization of the medical industry. In a world in which we had direct payment, bu-

---

20. See note 19.

reaucracy would be significantly reduced, competition among doctors and insurers would be promoted, many medical developments would be less expensive, and patients would control their health care system.

Clearly, patients must spend directly and consciously for health care; otherwise, considerations of cost will not enter into purchasing. The transaction must occur directly between patient and doctor rather than be shielded from free market effects by the third-party payer system. Let the free market "control" costs, just as it does in other service industries. Cost consciousness is vital to the workings of supply and demand. The structure of health care insurance needs to change to allow value-driven decisions and the control of money by patients. Reducing the restrictions on health savings accounts (including eligibility requirements) and promoting consumer education are areas in which government can play an important role. Improvements in quality and efficiency will also result from the value-driven purchasing of medical care. The U.S. population will welcome these empowering changes. The government just needs to trust the people with their own money.

Chapter Two

The Medical Liability System: Current Debates

Daniel P. Kessler

Introduction

Liability law allocates the costs of accidents among individuals. Accidental injuries are frequent in modern society. One car rear-ends another, damaging property and causing personal injury; a soda pop bottle explodes, injuring a consumer; a physician misdiagnoses a patient's illness, resulting in medical complications when the illness is ultimately treated.

Liability law has two principal goals. The first goal is to provide compensation to parties injured in accidents. The "compensation" goal of liability law attempts to provide a form of social insurance against accidental injuries. The second goal is to provide potential injurers with the incentive to avoid accidents for which the social cost of prevention is less than the cost created by the accident—that is, to induce the best possible deterrence. The "deterrence" goal of liability law is designed to induce individuals to internalize the nega-

The material in this essay is a revised version of "The Economic Effects of the Liability System" (Hoover Essay in Public Policy Number 91, 1998) and of "Tort Liability and the Patients' Bill of Rights," which appeared in the *Weekly Standard* of January 3/10, 2000.

tive externality created by engaging in careless behavior, by charging injurers for the accidents that they cause. If taking precaution against harming others is costly, and potential injurers are not required to pay for the harm that they cause, then they will in general take less precaution than is socially optimal; potential injurers will cause accidents that could have been prevented for less than the cost created by the accident.

In theory, by requiring people to pay compensation equal to the harm that they cause if an accident occurs, the law can induce potential injurers to take the efficient or socially optimal level of precaution—the level of precaution where the marginal cost of precaution equals the marginal benefit—by forcing them to internalize the externality.

In practice, however, the liability system serves neither goal well in markets for health care. The system has high transaction costs and fails to compensate injured parties appropriately. Only one in fifteen patients who suffer an injury due to medical negligence receives compensation, and five-sixths of the cases that receive compensation have no evidence of negligence.[1] Instead, the main determinant of whether an injury receives compensation is the extent of injury, not the extent of fault.[2] In addition, the system leads to inefficient precautionary care decisions by doctors and patients, or defensive medicine—precautionary treatments that have little medical benefit and are administered out of the fear of legal liability. Why does the medical liability system perform as poorly as it does? And which of the currently proposed policy reforms can help improve its functioning?

---

1. "Patients, Doctors, and Lawyers: Medical Injury, Malpractice Litigation, and Patient Compensation in New York," *Harvard Medical Practice Study* (Cambridge, MA: Harvard University Press, 1990); P. C. Weiler et al., *A Measure of Malpractice: Medical Injury, Malpractice Litigation, and Patient Compensation* (Cambridge, MA: Harvard University Press, 1993).

2. Troyen A. Brennan, C. M. Cox, and H. R. Burstin, "Relation between Negligent Adverse Events and the Outcomes of Medical Malpractice Litigation," *New England Journal of Medicine* 335:26 (December 26, 1996): pp. 1963–67.

In this essay, I evaluate the effects of three kinds of proposed reform: limits on liability, such as caps on noneconomic damages; expansion of liability to managed care plans, as in some versions of the "patients' bill of rights"; and other reforms, such as medical practice guidelines, alternative dispute resolution, and no-fault insurance.

The Source of the Problem in Medical Liability

In theory, doctors and patients trade off the benefits and costs of precautionary medical care. For example, suppose a diagnostic test costs $500 but gives patients an extra year of life with probability .01. If the patients value a year of life at $50,000 or more, then they and their physicians will undertake the test; but if the patients value a year of life at less than $50,000, then they will not.

In practice, however, doctors and patients only trade off the benefits against the costs of care that they bear directly. Because of health insurance, this generally accounts for a small part of the true total cost: the insured portion of expenses for drugs, tests, and medical services tends to be larger than the uninsured portion. In addition, although physicians are generally insured against the financial costs of malpractice, they are not insured against the substantial nonfinancial costs—including the harm to reputation, lowered self-esteem from adverse publicity, and time and unpleasantness of defending against a claim.

In this situation, even a liability system that functioned costlessly and awarded damages exactly equal to harm would lead doctors and patients to undertake precautionary treatments that had greater costs than benefits. The substantial transaction costs imposed by the liability system only increase the incentive to undertake low-benefit precautionary treatment. The combination of the adverse incentive effects of health insurance and the transaction costs of the liability system create an environment in which defensive medicine is the natural response.

Evaluating Proposed Policy Reforms

Limits on Liability

Previous research suggests that certain legal reforms that limit liability in medical care reduce the practice of defensive medicine. Table 2.1 lists eight common reforms to states' medical liability laws. The table categorizes these reforms in two groups, direct reforms and indirect reforms. Direct reforms include changes in laws that specify statutory limits or reductions in malpractice awards: caps on total or noneconomic damages, collateral source rule reforms (which require damages to be reduced by all or part of the dollar value of collateral source payments to the plaintiff), abolition of punitive damages, and mandatory prejudgment interest. Indirect reforms include changes that affect awards only indirectly, such as reforms imposing mandatory periodic payments (which require damages in certain cases to be disbursed in an annuity that pays out over time) and caps on attorneys' contingency fees, as well as the abolition of joint-and-several liability for total or noneconomic damages, creation of a patient compensation fund, and imposition of comparative negligence.

Table 2.2 compares the hospital expenditures and health of Medicare beneficiaries with severe cardiac illness in states with and without direct reforms. The table is based on the analysis of longitudinal data on all elderly Medicare recipients hospitalized for the treatment of a new heart attack, or acute myocardial infarction (AMI), or of new ischemic heart disease (IHD) in 1984, 1987, and 1990.[3] (Because AMI is essentially a more severe form of the same underlying illness as IHD is, we can assess whether reforms affect more or less severe cases of a health problem differently by comparing AMI with IHD patients.) We study the effect of the tort law reforms adopted from 1985 to 1990 on total hospital expenditures

---

3. Daniel P. Kessler and Mark B. McClellan, "Do Doctors Practice Defensive Medicine?" *Quarterly Journal of Economics* 111 (1996): pp. 353–390.

Table 2.1   Eight Common Reforms to States' Medical Liability Laws

Reform	Description of Reform	Potential Effect on Liability
Caps on damage awards	Either noneconomic (pain and suffering) or total damages payable are capped at a statutorily-specified dollar amount	Direct
Abolition of punitive damages	Medical malpractice defendants are not liable for punitive damages under any circumstances	Direct
No mandatory prejudgment interest	Interest on either noneconomic or total damages accruing from either the date of injury or the date of the filing of the lawsuit is not mandatory	Direct
Collateral source rule reform	Total damages payable in a malpractice tort are statutorily reduced by all or part of the dollar value of collateral source payments to the plaintiff	Direct
Caps on contingency fees	The proportion of an award that a plaintiff can contractually agree to pay a contingency-fee attorney is capped at a statutorily specified level	Indirect
Mandatory periodic payments	Part or all of damages must be disbursed in the form of an annuity that pays out over time	Indirect
Joint-and-several liability reform	Joint and several liability is abolished for noneconomic or total damages, either for all claims or for claims in which defendants did not act in concert	Indirect
Patient compensation fund	Doctors receive government-administered excess malpractice liability insurance, generally financed through a tax on malpractice insurance premiums	Indirect

Source: Kessler and McClellan, "Do Doctors Practice Defensive Medicine?"

Table 2.2 Hospital Expenditures and Mortality Outcomes, in States with and without Direct Reforms, for Elderly Medicare Beneficiaries with Heart Disease, 1984–1990

	1-Year Total Hospital Expenditures					1-Year Mortality				
	1984	1987	1990	1984–87 % Change	1984–90 % Change	1984	1987	1990	1984–87 % Change	1984–90 % Change
Patients Hospitalized for Heart Attack										
States without Direct Reforms	$10,194	$11,810	$12,618	15.9%	23.8%	40.2%	39.1%	35.7%	−1.1%	−4.5%
States with Direct Effect before 1985	$10,513	$11,722	$13,022	11.5%	23.9%	40.1%	39.0%	35.4%	−1.1%	−4.7%
States Enacting Direct Reforms Effective from 1985 to 1987	$11,304	$12,595	$13,186	11.4%	16.6%	39.5%	38.6%	35.3%	−0.9%	−4.2%
States Enacting Direct Reforms Effective from 1988 to 1990	$8,960	$9,865	$10,925	10.1%	21.9%	41.9%	39.2%	35.7%	−2.7%	−6.2%
Patients Hospitalized for Ischemic Heart Disease										
States without Direct Reforms	$9,439	$10,859	$12,083	15.0%	28.0%	14.1%	12.0%	11.0%	−2.1%	−3.1%
States with Direct Reforms in Effect before 1985	$10,331	$11,064	$12,505	7.1%	21.0%	13.5%	11.7%	10.7%	−1.8%	−2.8%
States Enacting Direct Reforms Effective from 1985 to 1987	$10,527	$11,315	$12,300	7.5%	16.8%	13.8%	11.6%	10.5%	−2.2%	−3.3%
States Enacting Direct Reforms Effective from 1988 to 1990	$9,241	$9,623	$11,421	4.1%	23.6%	14.1%	12.3%	11.5%	−1.8%	−2.6%

Note: Hospital expenditures in 1991 dollars. Source: Kessler and McClellan, "Do Doctors Practice Defensive Medicine?": Table 3.

on the patient in the year after AMI or IHD, to measure the intensity of treatment. We also model the effect of tort law reforms on important patient outcomes. We estimate the effect of reforms on a serious adverse outcome that is common in our study population: mortality within one year of the occurrence of cardiac illness.

The main hypothesis that we test is as follows. If reductions in medical malpractice tort liability lead to reductions in intensity but not to increases in adverse health outcomes, holding constant other state political and regulatory characteristics, then medical care for these health problems is defensive—that is, doctors supply a socially excessive level of care because of malpractice liability pressures. Put another way, tort reforms that reduce liability also reduce inefficiency in the medical care delivery system to the extent that they reduce health expenditures that do not provide commensurate benefits. We assess the magnitude of defensive treatment behavior by calculating the cost of an added year of life or an added year of cardiac health achieved through treatment intensity induced by specific aspects of the liability system. If liability-induced precaution results in low expenditure per year of life saved relative to generally accepted cost per year of life saved of other medical treatments, then the existing liability system provides incentives for efficient care; but if liability-induced precaution results in high expenditure per year of life saved, then the liability system provides incentives for socially excessive care.

The table reports conditional means for expenditure and mortality for patients from states adopting and not adopting direct reforms, unadjusted for patient demographic characteristics or other differences between states. The table reflects several well-known facts about the treatment of heart disease in the United States. Real resources spent on hospitalization for heart disease have grown dramatically everywhere in the United States. For example, expenditure for elderly patients with heart attacks grew from approximately 17 to 24 percent in real terms from 1984 to 1990, depending on the patient's state of residence. Coincident with this growth in resource use was a dramatic improvement in average mortality from heart disease. In 1984, an elderly American had approximately a 40 percent probability of dying within one year of suffering a heart attack; by 1990, although the population had aged slightly, the probability of dying within one year of a heart attack had fallen to approximately 35 percent—*fully a 12.5 percent decline in one-year mortality (.35– .40/.40), in only seven years.* Thus, the average expenditure-benefit ratio of the increased treatment for heart attack in the 1980s was approximately $50,000 per year of life saved.*

However, the *marginal* expenditure-benefit ratio of the *additional* increase in care attributable to high levels of medical malpractice liability pressure was much higher. As the table shows, patients from states without direct reforms experienced substantially greater growth in expenditures on heart disease without experiencing much greater rates of improvement in health outcomes, as compared with patients from adopting states. Expenditure growth was slower in the reform, compared with the nonreform, states for AMI, and trend differences were slightly greater for IHD. In contrast, mortality trends on average were quite similar for reform and nonreform states. These results suggest that doctors practice defensive medicine and that direct reform to the liability system improves productivity in health care by achieving reductions in resource use with no adverse effect on output, for example, patient health. These simple comparisons do not account for differences in trends in patient characteristics across the state groups, do not account for differences in the political and regulatory environments of states, and do not account for any effects of other potentially correlated reforms. Nonetheless, they anticipate the results that follow.

Figures 2.1 and 2.2 present regression-adjusted trends in hospital expenditures and patient health outcomes for elderly heart attack

---

*This figure is based on the average expenditure for AMI in 1984 of $10,881; average expenditure for AMI in 1990 of $13,140; average mortality in 1984 of 35.4 percentage points; and average mortality in 1990 of 39.9 percent. Thus the average expenditure-benefit ratio of incremental intensity supplied from 1984 to 1990 was equal to $(13,140 - 10,881)/(.399 - .354) = \$50,200$.

Figure 2.1 Regression-Adjusted Expenditures, Subsequent Illness, and Mortality in Elderly Heart Attack Patients in States with and without Direct Reforms

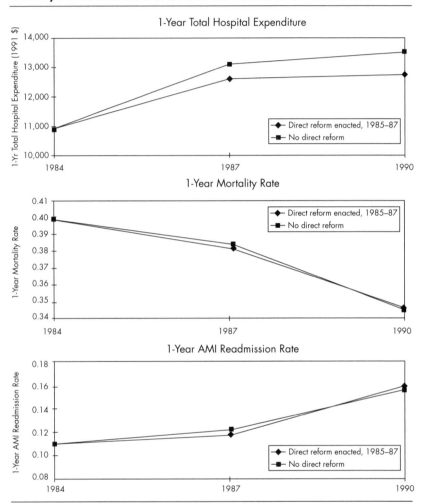

Source: Daniel P. Kessler, ''The Economic Effects of the Liability System,'' Hoover Institution Essays in Public Policy Number 91.

Figure 2.2   Regression-Adjusted Expenditures, Subsequent Illness, and Mortality in Elderly Ischemic Heart Disease Patients in States with and without Direct Reforms

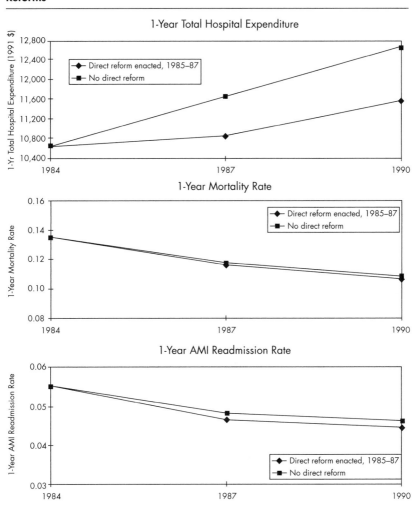

Source: Kessler, "The Economic Effects of the Liability System."

and ischemic heart disease patients (respectively) from states enacting a direct reform in the period from 1985 to 1987, compared with all other states. The figures present estimates of the effects of reform on two important health outcomes: subsequent illness (whether the patient experiences a later AMI requiring hospitalization in the year following the initial illness) and mortality. The trends in the two kinds of states coincide exactly in the first year because the levels of expenditures and health outcomes in the figures are calculated controlling for fixed differences across states, for time-varying state political and regulatory characteristics, and for patient demographic characteristics—patient age, gender, black or nonblack race, and urban or rural residence. These estimates also control for the presence of "indirect" reforms at the time of treatment and therefore isolate the effect of direct reforms on defensive practices.*

Figures 2.1 and 2.2 confirm that the simple descriptive statistics presented in table 2.2 are not an artifact of differences across states that are correlated with both direct reforms and medical treatment patterns. For example, the top panel of figure 1 shows that expenditure on heart attack treatment grew 7 percent more rapidly in states without direct reforms, as compared with states adopting direct reforms from 1985 to 1987; this difference was statistically significant at conventional levels. Mortality trends in these two groups, in contrast, were nearly identical and were not statistically distinguishable. As calculations in the 1996 article by Kessler and McClellan show, the expenditure-benefit ratio for a higher-pressure liability regime is more than $500,000 per additional one-year AMI survivor in 1991 dollars; even a ratio based on the upper bound of statistical confi-

---

*The estimates do not separately control for increase reforms because neither of the increase reforms is relevant to this study. The most common and important increase reform—comparative negligence—does not apply to medical malpractice cases (patients are never contributorily negligent). In addition, no state adopted or repealed prejudgment interest during the 1985–1990 study period.

dence intervals around the estimated effect of reform-induced treatment on mortality translates into hospital expenditures of more than $100,000 per additional AMI survivor to one year.[4] Results for outcomes related to quality of life—that is, rehospitalizations with recurrent AMI—also showed no consequential effects of reform.

Results for patients with IHD, presented in figure 2.2, are qualitatively similar to those just described for AMI. IHD expenditures also grew rapidly from 1984 to 1990. Direct reforms led to somewhat larger expenditure reductions for patients with IHD than with AMI, possibly reflecting the fact that IHD is a relatively less severe form of heart disease, for which more patients may have "marginal" indications for treatment. The effects of reforms on IHD outcomes are again very small. Thus direct liability reforms appear to have a relatively larger effect on the expenditure-benefit ratio of IHD treatments.

We estimated several additional models, discussed in detail in the 1996 article by Kessler and McClellan, to confirm the validity of these results. The main issue is whether differences in treatment between reform and nonreform states represent a true causal effect of reform or some other unmeasured difference between states. We estimated models controlling for statute-of-limitations reforms, to assess whether there were unobserved characteristics of states that were correlated with both the propensity to adopt legal reforms generally and medical treatment patterns, health care costs, and health outcomes. Statute-of-limitations reforms (which require that patients alleging injury file suit relatively sooner than has been traditionally required) should not have any effect on the treatment of elderly patients for heart disease because medical injury in this population is immediately apparent. We found that statute-of-limitations reforms had neither an economically nor statistically significant effect on expenditures and outcomes, consistent with the hypothesis

---

4. See note 3.

that these results were not biased by unobserved state-level factors that are correlated with direct reforms and health care decisions.

Patients' Bill of Rights

Would giving patients greater rights to sue their health plans lead to more appropriate care? Or would it lead to increased litigation, higher cost of treatment, and lower rates of health insurance coverage, without commensurate health benefits for patients?

These questions have been at the center of recent debates over the "patients' bill of rights." Current federal law, in the form of the Employee Retirement Income Security Act (Erisa) of 1974, has been interpreted as preempting most state law suits against health plans to recover damages for medical injuries. At the same time, Erisa sharply limits the plans' tort liability under federal law. Congress is considering expanding the patients' right to sue their plans, by reducing either the scope of Erisa's preemption of state tort law or Erisa's limitations on the plans' federal tort liability.

Unfortunately, because this expansion of liability for malpractice has no direct precedent, there is no hard evidence about its likely effects. (In existing state law, the expansions of plans' liability, such as those adopted by California, Georgia, Missouri, and Texas, are likely to have less dramatic consequences because their scope is limited by Erisa.)

The research above shows that incremental increases in malpractice liability lead to more defensive medicine. Recent work shows that this is true even in areas with high levels of managed care enrollment; more-parsimonious practices resulting from managed care's incentives have not fully eliminated defensive treatment behavior.[5]

To the extent that expanding liability for health plans increases

---

5. Daniel P. Kessler and Mark B. McClellan, "How Liability Reform Affects Medical Productivity," *Journal of Health Economics* 21 (2002): pp. 931–955.

malpractice liability, research suggests that it will lead to more waste-ful treatment. For example, more liability for plans could lead to more-frequent malpractice claims and more physician involvement with the liability system. Other work suggests that physicians would respond to these changes in incentives with costly increases in treat-ment intensity that yield few health benefits for patients.[6] But to the extent that expanding liability for plans shifts malpractice pressure from physicians to plans—and thereby decreases the pressure on physicians—it has the potential to reduce the cost of care and im-prove patients' well-being. Moreover, if plans have medical decision-making authority in practice, then it may enhance efficiency to real-locate tort liability from physicians to plans.

The devil is in the details. On the one hand, a patients' bill of rights that simply expands the number and complexity of malprac-tice suits has the potential to increase defensive medicine. On the other hand, a reform that lessens the malpractice pressure on physi-cians could lead to more efficient and effective medical care.

Other Reforms

Although direct reforms improve efficiency, they do little to improve the performance of the system in terms of the compensation goal. Caps on damages, for example, limit awards to those patients with the most serious injuries. For this reason, researchers and policymak-ers have suggested a wide range of largely untried reforms—some advocating radical changes to the allocation of responsibility for in-juries—that seek to address both compensation and deterrence goals. These reforms can be divided into three classes. The most gradual class of reforms retains the current system of trial by judge

6. Daniel P. Kessler and Mark B. McClellan, "Malpractice Law and Health Care Reform: Optimal Liability Policy in an Era of Managed Care," *Journal of Public Economics* 84 (2002): 175–197.

and jury but adds new guidelines or other structure to the legal process. Alternative dispute resolution (ADR), the second class of reforms, retains a fault-based system of allocating damages but replaces the traditional judicial system with mediation or arbitration. The most radical reforms propose no-fault insurance for injuries, often coupled with some administrative mechanism for allocating fault.

Guidelines

Guidelines are a commonly suggested mechanism for improving the process of resolving medical malpractice claims, although the general principle behind them could be extended to other kinds of tort claims. Medical practice guidelines specify appropriate treatments for patients in particular clinical circumstances. Guidelines would affect mainly the fourth element of a tort claim—the determination of negligence. Traditionally, physician negligence depends on a jury's finding of noncompliance with community standards of care, as interpreted by one or more expert witnesses. This relatively unstructured inquiry has the potential to lead to inconsistent or unpredictable application of the negligence rule.[7] Statutory reform to state liability law could allow defendants to use the compliance with practice guidelines to establish either an absolute or a rebuttable presumption of due care; conversely, guideline-based reforms could allow plaintiffs to use the noncompliance with guidelines to establish either an absolute or rebuttable presumption of negligence.

By systematizing the standard of care, guidelines may enable the liability system to process cases more quickly, more economically, and with fewer errors. In doing so, they may both improve compensation and reduce inefficient precautionary care. However, the design

---

7. Eleanor D. Kinney, "Malpractice Reform in the 1990s: Past Disappointments, Future Success?" *Journal of Health Politics, Policy, and Law* 20 (1995): pp. 99–135.

and implementation of a well-functioning system of guidelines is difficult. In health care, for example, *ex ante* specification of the relationship between illness and appropriate medical decision making would be at best extremely complex and would have to change rapidly with medical technology. Even the best-designed system of guidelines would most likely require expert testimony, case by case, to aid in interpretation and application.

Alternate Dispute Resolution

Under another proposal, states would replace the right to sue for certain kinds of injuries in tort with mandatory binding alternative dispute resolution (ADR), such as arbitration or mediation. ADR proposals generally transfer power to resolve claims into an administrative system with a specialized expert fact-finder and decision maker who operates under fewer constraints than civil court judges do. In this way, the goals of ADR are similar to those of guidelines: to provide a more rapid and accurate means of delivering compensation and apportioning responsibility for injury. ADR may offer substantial promise. But to the extent that an ADR system seeks to preserve all the evidentiary and due process rights that the parties would have in a tort case, it would be less likely to offer substantial advantages.

No-fault

No-fault systems are the most radical suggestion for the reform of the liability system. No-fault would also limit or remove patients' right to sue for certain injuries and instead compensate them according to a schedule of damages, an administrative hearing, or both, generally at a more modest level than occurs in tort, regardless of the fault of the alleged injurer. Most no-fault proposals are coupled with an additional administrative system that seeks to monitor the behavior of potential injurers, to preserve incentives for appropriate accident avoidance.

A well-functioning no-fault system offers the obvious advantage of improving compensation and reducing transaction costs. But our experience with automobile no-fault insurance systems suggests two serious drawbacks. The first is their expense—arising from no-fault's goal of compensating everyone who is injured rather than just those injured negligently. Indeed, the expense of a no-fault system is proportional to its success in compensating injured parties, particularly the severely injured. One response to this is to compensate only less severely injured parties through the no-fault system and to allow more severely injured parties to sue in tort. Many states have adopted limited no-fault approaches to compensating people injured in automobile accidents. However, although limiting the reach of a no-fault system may reduce its costs of operation, it would also reduce its benefits.[8] The second drawback to no-fault systems is that they eliminate the beneficial deterrence of the tort system. Empirical research in law and economics largely finds that automobile no-fault systems lead to increases in the fatal accident rate, with some earlier papers finding no effect.[9]

---

8. Stephen J. Carroll et al., "No-Fault Approaches to Compensating People Injured in Auto Accidents," Rand Report R-4019-ICJ. See especially chapter 4 for discussion.

9. Daniel P. Kessler and Daniel Rubinfield, "Empirical Study of the Civil Justice System" in *Handbook of Law and Economics*, ed. A. Mitchell Polinsky and Steven Shavell (Amsterdam: North Holland Publishers, forthcoming).

Chapter Three

The Realities of the Growth in Medical Spending

Mark V. Pauly

Introduction

Spending on medical care in the United States has grown in real terms, year in and year out, for as far back as we have data. Although there are brief periods of modest differences, growth has been very similar for private and public sector spending over the long term. The woefully misnamed "health care cost inflation" is usually cited as a major reason for the need to make fundamental changes in the health care system. (It is misnamed because the data do not measure cost and the reason for growth is not inflation.) Is the growth in this category of consumer spending a prima facie reason for concluding that current arrangements are deficient so that changes capable of producing improvement (by some definition) are needed? Are we even sure that it is an improvement to slow spending growth? I will attempt to help answer these questions by undertaking two tasks: first, to explain, at several levels, the reasons why real medical spending has increased; and second, to offer such evidence as exists on the normative judgment of whether increased spending for those reasons implies that there are feasible reforms that can improve matters. That is, I want to discuss whether the effects of higher real spending are negative for some or all of the population and, if they are, whether there is something that could and should be done about it.

What Do We Measure and What Do the Data Show?

I will rely on the "official" measures of medical spending provided by the Center for Medicare and Medicaid Studies' Division of National Cost [sic] Estimates.[1] According to these data, expenditures on per capita personal health care in both nominal and real (deflated by the gross domestic product [GDP] deflator) terms has almost always grown but at varying rates. As figure 3.1 shows, total real spending growth rates have historically fluctuated substantially around a trend of 3 to 4 percent a year. The figure also shows that the upsurge beginning in 1999, far from being atypical, is in the range of previous fluctuations and generally repeats the conventional pattern of high growth. Only the most recent (2002) data are much above trend (although there have been many such observations before) and that is due to some extent to a dramatic drop in the general price index (to 1.1 percent annually). There is nothing in these data to indicate that the current period is unusual, and evidence is starting to accumulate that spending growth is headed down again, judging from the recent results for two large private insurers (Aetna and Cigna) and from the demonstrated slowdown in hospital spending growth beginning in 2003.[2] Even so, real growth at 4 percent gener-

---

1. K. Levit et al., "Health Spending Rebound Continues in 2002," *Health Affairs* 23 (January/February 2004): 147–159.

2. P. B. Ginsburg, "Hospital Spending," *Health Affairs* 23 (January/February 2004): 273; B. C. Strunk and P. B. Ginsburg, "Tracking Health Care Costs: Trends Slow in First Half of 2003," *Center for Studying Health System Change Data Bulletin* 26 (December 2003).

Figure 3.1   Real Annual Rates of Total National Health Expenditure Growth Per Capita, 1961–2001

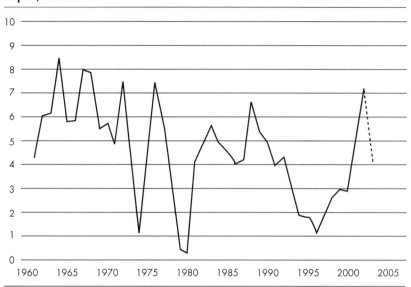

2003 data (shown in dashed line) based on the CMS projections; the CPI growth is estimated at 2 percent.

ally exceeds real growth in GDP so that the ratio of medical spending to measured GDP generally rises.

Some policymaker comments on these data: "Personal health care spending" differs from "national health expenditures" mainly in excluding the difference between insurer premiums and benefits, which in turn represents both insurer administrative expense and insurer profit. Spending estimates are based on the estimates of revenue flows gathered from various sources so that there is some error in measurement; although the magnitude of total spending is probably accurate, the estimate of changes in any one pair of years for any specific expenditure item is not totally reliable (and is in fact often revised after the release of data). A blip of 1 percent in the measured growth of spending may not be real. The measure of private insurance benefits (and premiums) is probably one of the least reliable numbers.

Some economist comments on the data: These are the measures of *revenue* received for medical goods and services; they are *not* the measures of cost to the economy. The revenue goes in large part to cover the true (opportunity) costs of the inputs used to produce those products, but it also goes to profits (for firms) and rents (for health personnel). Thus, if spending rises because more smart young people are drawn from doing other useful tasks in the economy into providing medical care, the real opportunity cost that the country as a whole pays is positive and equals the value of those other foregone tasks. In contrast, if spending rises because drug company profits or nurses' wages rise, with no change in the number working, those suppliers gain what consumers lose; the cost does not change, and the only effect is a transfer among Americans. This distinction between costs and transfers will be important later.

Why does spending rise? There are several ways to seek clues to answers to this question. One way is to see to whom the additional money goes, who receives it. Another is to see what (if anything) the additional money buys. A third is to see why people choose to buy those things. I will pursue all three strategies in this paper and then try to put the clues together to yield both explanation and evaluation.

Decomposing the Growth in Spending

It is traditional to try to decompose the growth in spending into two parts: the growth in input prices and returns (including changes in the profit on equity capital and rents on inputs in limited supply) and the residual (which is left over). The residual captures any change in the quantity of care (of various kinds), any change in the quality and kinds of care, demographic changes that influence the quantity of care demanded, and any change in the technical efficiency of production. It also represents payments to added inputs rather than just higher payments for inputs that were already there.

Figure 3.2 shows this decomposition for recent years for total health care; table 3.1 provides the basic data.

Some recent data on hospital spending (in table 3.1 and figure 3.3) may help illustrate what typically goes on and what inferences we can draw about it. There is a little drama here: hospital spending is the largest single share of total medical spending, but for most of the past decade it has grown at rates much lower than total medical spending. Then, suddenly and surprisingly, in the late 1990s hospital spending growth reawakened, at least for a while. What do we know about what happened and who got the money?

One way to view the growth in hospital spending is in terms of the "uses" of the added funds that spending represents. More than 60 percent of hospital spending is for labor, and a substantial fraction of its allocation to other services, such as laundry and prepared foods, represents the labor of workers, although workers not directly employed by the hospital. In contrast, direct capital expense for the plant and equipment is generally less than 10 percent of hospital accounting costs. Finally, payments for profits (for investor-owned

Figure 3.2 Shares of Real NHE Growth

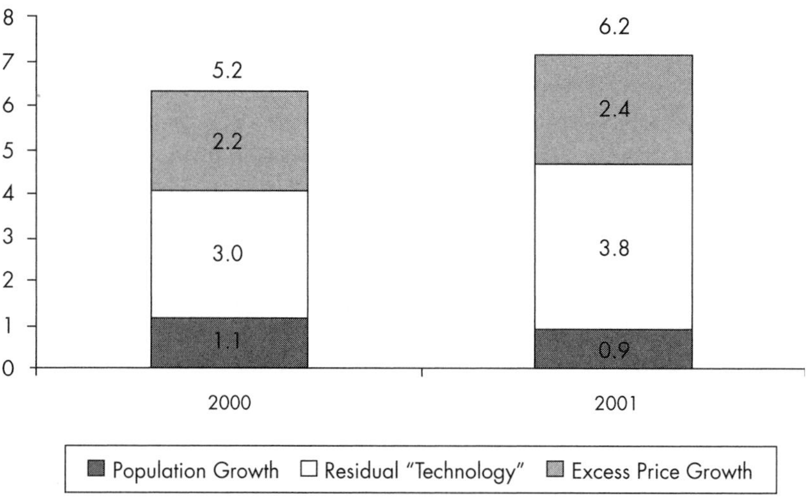

Table 3.1 Health Care Spending and Employment: Annual Rates of Growth

	1999	2000	2001	2002
ALL NHE				
Nominal NHE	5.7	7.4	8.5	9.3
Nominal PHE	5.2	6.9	8.5	8.8
NHE Deflated by GDP Deflator	4.2	5.2	6.0	8.1
NHE Deflated by HC Price	2.8	3.9	4.8	NA
NHE Deflated by HC wages	2.6	3.0	3.6	NA
Employment (FTE) (Health Services)	0.6	1.9	3.4	2.9
Private Hospital				
Nominal Spending Rev.	5.8	7.1	10.4	10.0
Nominal Spending Exps.	4.3	6.5	9.7	9.8
Spending Deflated by GDP Def.	3.3	4.9	7.8	7.4
Spending Deflated by ECI	2.6	3.0	4.7	4.6
Adj. Days	1.6	8.1	2.2	1.8
Employment (FTE)	1.1	0.4	2.9	3.3

NHE: National Health Expenditure; PHE: Personal Health Expenditures; GDP: Gross Domestic Product; HC: Health Care; FTE: Full-Time Equivalent; ECI: Employment Cost Index.

Figure 3.3 Shares of Real Hospital Revenue Growth

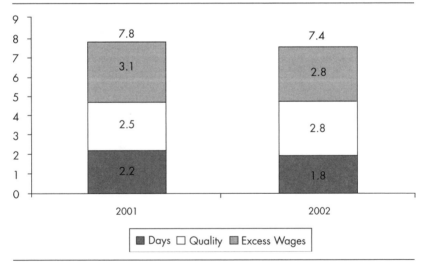

hospitals) or net revenues (for nonprofits) are only a tiny fraction of the total, never even approaching 5 percent. So, in a rough sense, this change in hospitals' spending can be broken down into three parts: the change in (mostly labor) input prices, the change in the volume of inputs (again, mostly labor), and the change in net income (profit). If we use the average (hours adjusted) change in wage rates as a rough measure of input prices, figure 3.3 shows the decomposition of spending growth into these categories.

What are the normative implications of each? The change in wage rates is easiest to characterize: it represents (in the short run) a transfer to labor that might be related to a change in labor's opportunity cost (wages available elsewhere). This is not necessarily a cost to the economy, or at least not as large an increase in true cost as is the increase in spending. The change in labor quantity definitely has a cost: the cost is the value of the output that new labor could have produced if it were used elsewhere. Finally, the interpretation of the change in net income depends on the kind of hospital ownership. If it is investor-owned, higher profits are a transfer to investors. If it is nonprofit, the questions are what those profits will be used for and what the value of that use is.

A significant fraction (but less than half) of the recent growth in household spending is a transfer from consumers to hospital workers. How this transfer is evaluated depends in large part on who one thinks is more deserving of higher real income. However, if the reason for rising wages is a larger quantity of labor demand pressing on a more or less fixed supply curve, such normative judgments may not matter much; no one would want to deny higher wages to nurses just because there was a shortage of nurses. Higher transfers to stockholders (profits) might be viewed differently in the average person's value judgment, but the net income of hospitals is generally not a large part of rising spending, as it was not in these years. The category of spending most relevant for a normative judgment about efficiency is the approximately 60 percent of spending growth accounted for by hiring more workers.

The main economic question is not one that most people would ask. It is not whether these hospital workers "need" jobs or whether they are getting better jobs (for which the answer is yes on both counts) but whether whatever these new workers will be doing in hospitals is of greater value to all consumers than whatever else the workers would have been doing. Obviously, if the new workers do not enhance either the quantity or the quality of hospital output, this is pure waste: any positive cost for something useless is wasteful. If there is unemployment, or unionization, it may be hard to know what the true opportunity cost of these workers is. If the workers do increase output or quality, the question is one of the value of that output.

For total health care spending, figure 3.2 gives much the same story. Excess (over economy-wide) price growth represents a significant fraction of spending growth but is less than that attributable to the residual "technology."

From the viewpoint of the welfare of all Americans, the changes in wages, prices, or profits are largely zero-sum. Since almost all inputs into health care are produced with American labor (this is true even of many nominally "foreign" drug firms that do the bulk of their research and production in the United States), the only difference transfers make to the economy is whether the donor or receiver saves and invests more, thus fostering growth in total national income. In contrast, the analysis of the desirability of drawing yet more labor into this sector turns on relative valuation, a subject to be discussed in more detail below. Finally, the desirability of higher "nonprofit profits" also depends on the comparison of benefits with opportunity cost, a comparison often to the disadvantage of nonprofit hospitals.[3] The usual resource misallocation that arises when

---

3. S. Nicholson et al., "Measuring Community Benefits Provided by For-Profit and Nonprofit Hospitals," *Health Affairs* 19 (November/December 2000): 168–177.

prices exceed marginal cost is likely to be relatively small because medical demand is inelastic and insurance is present.

What Kind of Output Do We Get?

So the reality is that the bulk of medical spending growth represents new resources flowing into this sector, associated with a statistical residual that we label (for want of better information) "technology" or "quality." If more inputs are diverted to the medical care sector, what do they do? In the hospital example, we have a rough-and-ready measure of quantity in the form of "adjusted" patient days (in which outpatient visits are converted into inpatient day equivalents based on relative prices[4]). We can then divide the change in spending in a different way: into a change in quantity and (as a residual) a change in what is literally input intensity per unit of output, often called "quality" (but that could also be called "new waste," depending on what the inputs went for). As the table shows, controlling for input prices, this "quality" measure is more important than quantity and quantity and quality together are more important than wages. As luck would have it, however, this quality is hard to measure and even harder to evaluate.

Several categories in this component are possible and are used (often inconsistently) by analysts. First, there may be changes in staffing required by regulation or undertaken in response to a perceived greater malpractice threat. Of course, such regulatory-compulsory sources do not preclude the possibility that the quality change is highly valuable. Indeed, such an assumption would be nearly a necessity if the regulation or liability were itself to be desirable.

Next, there may be "new technologies" in the commonsense

---

4. For instance, if the average charge for a visit is one-tenth the average charge per day, ten visits equal one day.

view of new patented inventions. Most entries in this category are pharmaceutical, but there can also be new devices (coated stents) or instruments (lasers). Yet if the technology itself is at first embodied in a physical product, or piece of equipment, its contribution to employment growth often depends on its use of complementary labor.

But the use of labor in new ways (without new machines or tools) to produce more effective output may also represent new technology. For example, the hiring of discharge planners whose advice improves patients' postdischarge quality of life represents a change in the way inputs are applied to output.

The real controversy arises with the valuation of this technology. Cost-benefit and cost-effectiveness analyses could establish this value but are presently limited in what they can do and how seriously they are taken. They have an especially hard time if the benefit is positive but small relative to the cost, exactly the "close calls" that might be debated as things that should or should not be done. As before, some of the evaluation will apply to the question of whether to use a new technology at all, and some will apply to how intensively it should be used, in the aggregate, and in patients with specific characteristics. I will further review below what (little) we know about the answer to the valuation question.

A second approach to decomposing spending growth is to attribute it to specific causes. The easiest call to make here concerns the effect of population. Population growth, which occurs these days at annual rates of 1 percent or even a little less, should (one might assume) increase spending by an equal percentage amount. Another commonly cited cause is the change in the age distribution of the population. As the population ages, that would seem to call for higher levels of spending. The actual annual magnitude of this effect at present is small, only about one-half of 1 percent or less. However, if we compare geographic areas (countries, states, counties) with varying proportions of older people, there is no strong evidence that a larger proportion of older people is associated with a higher level of spending or use. So while the old always use more care than the young do, apparently the system as a whole sometimes makes a downward adjustment in the average spending level at all ages to offset increases in the proportion of older people. The process by which this happens is a mystery.

Even if we adjust for these demographic changes, we can account for at most about 1.5 percent of real medical spending growth. Taking out the 2 percent due to higher input prices, that leaves about 2 to 2.5 percent a year as a residual, representing (definitionally) "more real inputs per capita, age adjusted." What is this, and what is it worth?

The usual explanation, and the one I generally agree with, is that this residual reflects the costly but beneficial new technology already mentioned. But there is no necessity that such technology be invented or, if it is, that it be adopted or, if it is adopted, that it take so costly a form. That is, consumers need not necessarily demand this new technology just because it has been invented. Why do they do so, and why do they do so to the extent that they do? Whatever the value of costly new technology, why do consumers (and insurers on their behalf) demand it and then pay for it?

We have only some crude answers to these questions. At the most fundamental level, it is clear that human beings seek to live longer lives with high physical quality of life. Avoiding death, discomfort, disability, and even disfigurement is a good for which people are willing to pay the cost, that is, to sacrifice other goods that they value. But the fact that there is a high demand for health, broadly defined, only means that people will spend money on medical care, not that they will spend more money every year.

But they may be induced to spend more in the current year if there is a change in technology that allows them to buy additional health at a lower price than was available in the previous year. And if the demand for health is sufficiently price elastic, they may spend more in total at this lower price.

Take the extreme case of a serious disease (e.g., multiple sclerosis or Alzheimer's) that is initially untreatable in any serious way. One could say that the price of improving health is infinite, or nearly so. When the price is so high, people choose to spend nothing. The marginal value benefit or value from prospective improvement in health is quite high, but the price is higher still; there is no point in spending anything. Now let technology invent (as it has) a moderately effective treatment, perhaps one that only slows the progression of the disease. People may prefer to spend for this treatment (rather than for other things), and, if the treatment is a patented product, the price they will be charged will be high if their marginal valuation is high. If the technological change is effective enough, and if there is no patent protection, new technology can help spending fall: this has been the case for infectious diseases like polio and syphilis. But the patented "halfway" technologies (to use the term suggested by Lewis Thomas) that we usually see invented are not of this kind. And if technology cuts the cost per unit of treating a disease but also substantially improves the quality, the effect of higher quality may so increase the quality demanded that total spending rises. We think that is the case for laparoscopic surgery, at least initially.[5]

I think that these ideas help answer a question (and implicit criticism) of technological change in health care that is often posed. "Why is it," critics want to know, "that technological change reduces cost for things like computers and chicken but not for medical services?" One answer is that the demand for the underlying "commodity" people seek is less price elastic for these other things; I do not want that much more food because it is cheaper, but I do want more health if its price falls from infinity. That certainly seems true for the quantity of foodstuffs (as distinct from the quality, which may not always be improved by hybridization or factory farming). The other answer is that some of those changes represent the "full

---

5. A. P. Legorreta et al, "Increased Cholecystectomy Rate after the Introduction of Laparoscopic Cholecystectomy," *Journal of the America Medical Association* (September 22, 1993); 270 (12): 1429–1432.

way" technology, which reduces the price of doing almost anything to something close to zero, as is the case with the PC-Internet combination.

The economist William Baumol has provided another explanation.[6] He argues that, relative to manufacturing and agriculture, the possibilities for improving productivity in services like health care are more limited. The rising productivity in those other sectors, translated into higher economy-wide wages, means that the relative prices of services will rise. If demand is inelastic, total spending and the share of measured GDP will rise too. We could have a lower rate of growth in medical spending, by this argument, if we could squelch productivity improvements elsewhere in the economy.

So what is the value of new technology? The work of Cutler and McClellan and others is definitive here: for expenses for heart and circulatory disease, the benefit in the money value of improved health dwarfs the increase in real cost.[7] It even exceeds by a substantial margin the increase in total spending. Higher spending is "worth it" in that case.[8] But we do not know the aggregate value of spending increases for all diseases. More important, we do not know whether we would have gotten 80 percent of the benefit for 20 percent of the cost, and then whether the remaining 20 percent of the benefit was worth its cost.

What Will Happen to Spending Growth?
Will It Continue to Explode?

The current rate of real growth in medical spending resumes the pattern and level that occurred before the managed care transition in

---

6. W. J. Baumol, "Macroeconomics of Unbalanced Growth: The Anatomy of Urban Crisis," *The American Economic Review* 57 (June 1967): 415–426.

7. D. Cutler et al., "Pricing Heart Attack Treatments," in *Medical Care Output and Productivity*, ed. D. Cutler and E. Berndt (Chicago: University of Chicago Press, 2001), 305–362.

8. D. Cutler and M. McClellan, "Is Technological Change in Medicine Worth It?" *Health Affairs* (September/October 2001): 11–29.

the mid-1990s. The public sector rate has been lower largely because Medicare does not cover prescription drugs. The overall rate is close to the rate for earlier periods, although there is considerable fluctuation. At least it is in a range that we have often seen before. At this level, there is nothing new. Its slight excess also has a precedent: periods of low growth are usually matched with equally long periods of unusually high growth. In short, at the level of aggregate data, it appears to be business as usual, not the end of the world.

One place with much above-average growth appears to be private health insurance. This insurance (in contrast to Medicare) does cover costs for outpatient prescription drugs, and those costs are growing at a rate that has receded considerably from its 1999 peak but is still above average.

The year 2002 is the last for which we have actual official aggregate data, but some more current data have recently raised sustained concern. One is the answers employers give to surveys asking about their projected health benefits costs. Few employers covered by risk-bearing insurers will pay the premium charged, although experience rating means that there could be reductions or add-ons next year based on what actually happens. But the bulk of employees are covered by self-insured plans, whose insurance costs cannot be known until the year is over and claims have all come in. Employers may change coverage or insurers to reduce actual costs. So I expect actual premiums to rise by less than the 12 to 13 percent that has been forecasted and to continue to slow for the next five years, as does the official estimate provided by the Centers for Medicare and Medicaid Services (CMS).

The most reasonable projection, I believe, is that medical care will continue to take a bite out of increases in the economy's productivity and the citizens' real income that is moderately disproportionate to the growth in income, but surely not so much so that the growth in income spendable on other things will decline.[9] A rough

---

9. D. Cutler, M. Chernew, and R. Hirth, "Increased Spending on Health Care: How Much Can the United States Afford?" *Health Affairs* 22 (July/August 2003): 15–25.

calculation from relatively recent data is that the "marginal propensity to spend" an increase in total compensation on health care is about 0.2.[10] That is, the average American who gets a 5 percent raise seems to want to spend about 1 percent of that on medical care. At least for the foreseeable future, then, medical care spending will grow in real terms at a moderately rapid rate and the share of GDP (and productive imports) being used for medical care will grow modestly, topping out at around 20 percent. Things won't go on like this forever.

What we do not know, however, is the vehicle by which this slowdown will be brought about (nor do we expect that it will proceed in a tidy fashion). What we do know is that the growth that nevertheless does materialize will be, on balance, a good thing, representing choices by rational people to take a large minority of their increased real income in the form of enhanced quantity and quality of life. Health will be chosen over potatoes, shirts, and even housing because additions to it are valued more than what the same money could buy, or the same resources could do, if applied to something else.

The problem then is not the prospect of this kind of medical spending growth. I believe it is feasible, proper, and rational. It represents, on average, value for money. The problem rather is assuring ourselves that this is true. We would like to believe that real spending growth on medical care is worth it, but how can we get over the nagging doubt that it is not? People have the feeling that the usual test of value for money is lacking. For almost all products, the fact that someone was willing to pay the price means that the product is worth the price. But the presence of health insurance breaks this easy equivalency for health care. If I get an MRI (magnetic resonance imaging) or a bottle of pills for my migraine headaches, which the insurance pays for, there is no basis for concluding that they are

---

10. M. V. Pauly, "Should We Be Worried about High Real Medical Spending Growth in the United States?" *Health Affairs Web Exclusive*, January 8, 2003, http://www.healthaffairs.org/WebExclusives/2201Pauly.pdf.

worth as much to me as they cost, or indeed that they are worth much *at all*.

Insurers in principle have an alternative way of assuring value for money. If a newly insured product, in total, will cost more to consumers (through higher premiums) than it is worth, the unregulated insurer will refuse to cover.[11] Life is more complex if the new technology provides large benefits to some and unequivocally positive but small benefit to others. It is then much harder for insurers to titrate or ration the product to be consistent with such differences in benefits. The line of least resistance, once the door is open, is to make the technology available to all patients for whom physicians expect a positive benefit. Obviously, it would be ideal to limit this low-value use, and a variety of devices, from patient cost sharing to clinical guidelines, can do so, even if only imperfectly. But if the excess of cost over benefit for the low-benefit people (subject to the best method of constraining this "moral hazard") exceeds the positive net benefit to the high-benefit people, the competitive insurer (unconstrained by state laws or mandates) will again refuse to cover. Thus we get a very strong result.[12] If insurers do choose to cover a new technology (compared with not having it covered at all), that technology must be efficient, in the sense that the benefit from the technology and the risk reduction benefit from insurance coverage (taken together) must exceed the cost or additional premium associated with the technology. *There cannot be an excessively high or excessively costly rate of technical change* in competitive insurance and medical care markets.

But, you may object, how can we afford this new technology? Yogi Berra famously remarked (of a restaurant in which he worked in the off-season), "it's so crowded nobody goes there anymore." In a

---

11. M. V. Pauly, "Market Insurance, Public Insurance, and the Rate of Technological Change in Medical Care," *The Geneva Papers on Insurance and Risk* 28 (April 2003): 180–193.

12. Pauly, "Market Insurance."

similar logical view, one could complain that drug companies, hospitals, and doctors "are making so much money from health care that nobody can afford to buy it anymore." The pedantic point is that high spending must be made by, and therefore afforded by, at least *some* consumers. Once (or if) consumers decide they can't "afford" the latest new technology, they won't buy it anymore. Then either spending will not occur or (more plausibly, especially for patented drugs) the price will be dropped to a level consumers are willing to pay.

So, to state it simply, one cannot assert that higher spending on new technology is hurting the average consumer, compared with a situation in which the technology did not exist. It should be providing benefits greater than costs by a large amount. Then what is the problem? Why did we instinctively cringe when we heard that real spending growth in 2002 was higher than in 2001? Of course, consumers would rather pay less for what they get, but that would not affect efficiency, only distribution. I think there are two possible problems. One possibility is that, even if the new technology we bought in 2002 for an extra $190 billion was worth it (compared with sticking to the 2001 technology), it could be that we could have gotten 90 percent of that benefit for much less than 90 percent of the cost. That is, there might still be a lot of waste at the margin that somebody should do something about.

The other possibility is that the technology that many can afford may be overpriced for some who react by dropping insurance coverage or quietly going bankrupt. But why should this step be necessary? Usually, the old cheaper technology is still available: you can still obtain aspirin, noncoated stents, and oat bran rather than Imitrex, drug-eluting stents, and statins. It should be possible to keep the old technology in place; its price is less clear but probably need not rise even as much as overall health input prices. And the people for whom the added value of the latest technology is less than the added cost should prefer a "Classic Care Insurance," which covers the old but not the new, to no insurance at all. The availability of charity care also influences private insurance purchase, but its effect is small and especially so for the growing number of definitely not-poor uninsured. Why then is demand for insurance as sensitive to quality-related spending and premium growth as it appears to be?

I think this is a major puzzle and problem. One can think of excuses. While old technologies may still be available, doctors or lawyers may be uncomfortable about people using them. Consumers may not know how to find insurance that specializes in this care, and insurers may not know how to market coverage that isn't as good as it could be but is cheap. Employers may also not feel comfortable offering intentionally inferior options, and editorial page writers will be bound to jump on anyone who does. But the alternative of the best or nothing at all seems even less attractive.

The relationship of insurance to the valuation of new technology has two dimensions. Let us suppose that the valuation of a technology depends on income and illness severity and each person (at any point in time) will use one unit. If the distribution of illness is independent of income and if the value of the technology rises with income, given severity, then both the value and the rate of use of the technology will differ by income.

A compromise strategy would be to offer insurance with patient cost sharing to low-income people only, since they will ideally use less than high-income people will. This insurance will be a better deal for them than either full-coverage insurance (which they may use at the same rate but value the use less) or insurance pooled with higher-income people where the premium is biased upward by the higher use of higher-income people.

More generally, I would blame a kind of "money illusion." I see the money cost of my insurance rise by $50 a month, but I cannot see so clearly the new technology that money buys. And my employer sees this even less clearly. Price increases are certain; quality increases are contingent and imprecise. Closing this information gap appears to be important.

Where Will It All Go?

The *percentage rate* of spending growth eventually has to be brought down below the levels it has reached in recent years, but the absolute increase in real spending can remain high and the rate of growth can remain above that of real income. The bulk of Americans who are insured and not elderly have been experiencing spending growth, and that group almost surely has been made better-off by spending more on something of great average value. For that group, the worst thing that could happen would be for spending growth to slow down, because this would mean that the opportunities of increasing the length and quality of life had diminished; they would only have more mundane things to spend additional real income on. My own forecast is a modest tailing off of this growth, but no great rejoicing by chief financial officers.

For those of us who are or will soon be eligible for the tax-financed Medicare program, I think that things are more ominous. It is not that the middle class who now predominate among the elderly will value technical change less after their sixty-fifth birthday than they did before; it is rather that the vehicle through which they may express that valuation will become more sluggish and they will be forced to raise money in costly and unpopular ways. Specifically, higher taxes for Medicare mean higher distortion or higher "excess burden" on the economy. Trying to get a frugal government to raise the taxes of a shrinking and skeptical young work force is not a challenge I personally relish; I think it is a recipe for intense political conflict and confusion. Thus the main message here is that what the nonelderly insured can handle with relative equanimity will pose extraordinarily difficult financial problems for the Medicare program, difficulties that will be accentuated if drug coverage is added.

Conversely, the kind of spending growth my cohort will demand when we go on Medicare will seriously discomfort our grandchildren, who will largely need to pay for it. I don't know what will happen, but I am sure that efficiency and rationality will suffer. Medicare suffers more severe financial problems because it is by nature political and because it *raises* revenue through distortive taxes on non-beneficiaries. This means that it ought efficiently to do less, but politically it cannot admit to doing so.

The other group for which there will potentially be a problem is the near poor and the "near uninsured." For some reasons described above and for more reasons that we do not understand, some people seem to overreact to rising insurance premiums that pay for new technology, by bailing out of private insurance entirely. Some of these dropouts are almost totally irrational: they are workers who take jobs (with lower wages) where coverage is offered, and then they reject coverage because of employee premiums that are only a small fraction of the average value of benefits, and do this even if they are at high risk and very likely to need care.[13] They may say (and do say) that they can't "afford" the premiums, but then how can they afford out-of-pocket payments? Begging for free care or going without cannot be an attractive option.

The most plausible explanation is that the people who drop insurance are making a mistake, underestimating the need for, or the benefits of, insurance, and, most especially, underestimating the increase in the *value* of insurance that accompanies a quality-driven increase in premiums. Methods to communicate this value should be developed; that is, consumers should be informed that insurance benefits are valuable. One way to convey this message would be to describe explicitly why premiums rise and what they buy. People

---

13. L. J. Blumberg and L. M. Nichols, "The Health Status of Workers Who Decline Employer-Sponsored Insurance," *Health Affairs* 20 (November/December 2001): 180–187.

should be encouraged to purchase coverage; those who fail to do so should be treated as mistaken, not pitiful.

More specifically, what is needed is a clear statement of something individual insurance consumers, who are generally not sick, have a hard time seeing: that the new technologies have improved effects on the quality of life and survival, which consumers could obtain if they needed them. Perceptions probably lag most behind reality when and if both spending growth and improved technology accelerate simultaneously. A similar step would be public service campaigns intended to persuade people not to drop insurance. Rather than spend millions trying to persuade taxpayers to subsidize people who are confused, we should provide the potentially uninsured with information on how inexpensive insurance can be relative to the possible bills they would experience without it or to the benefit they would have to forego without it.

Another positive step would be to design and approve a less costly insurance plan than the low-deductible, low-copayment plans that well-off and well-subsidized consumers obtain. One could begin with a policy with coverage equivalent to today's Medicare: almost no drug, mental health, or preventive care coverage; a large inpatient deductible; and an upper limit on hospital days. Although such limited coverage would violate regulations in many states, Medicare coverage is customarily accepted to be part of a popular program. The Medicare limits would pare a lot off the premium for the average private policy. Moreover, the absence of drug coverage means that Medicare has avoided much of the source of the most rapid increases in private premiums.[14]

Another step that might improve insurance affordability and lower spending growth would be to remove or limit the current $100 billion (and more) subsidy to employment-based insurance. This

---

14. R. Pear, "Health Spending Rises to 15 Percent of Economy, a Record Level," *The New York Times*, January 8, 2004, sec. A, 15.

would surely produce a one-time but large reduction in spending, probably of about 10 to 15 percent, and that alone would bring back many of those lower-middle-income people who have dropped coverage. More speculatively, but perhaps more importantly, reducing coverage across the board might cause physician practice patterns to become more frugal. In addition, a lower level of coverage might stimulate a reduction in the rate of growth of spending, at least for a while. People with more frugal coverage would also presumably use less of any new technology offered for sale. At least initially, that would lower the rate of growth as well as the absolute amount of growth. The period of lower-growth rates would end when the base level of spending shrank.

A common suggestion to make insurance more affordable is to preclude state-mandated benefit laws that increase the premium for individual and small group insurance. There is some question about how much this would improve insurance take-up rates (since the lower premiums are offset by lower benefits). If there is an increase in take-up, that will provide strong evidence that the mandates are inefficient, adding more to premiums than to value.

Finally, generous subsidies to lower-middle-income people are needed in any case. That they would help those at the margin afford new, as well as old, technology is a point in their favor.

Conclusion

Perhaps most important, health policymakers should level with people. They should admit that it is almost impossible to lower cost without lowering quality, and that new information technology, managed care, malpractice reform, focused factories, medical savings accounts, chronic care management, or continuous quality improvement plans can produce at best little more than a small and temporary slowdown in the rates of spending growth. People should also be told as taxpayers to expect to pay higher premiums if they want to maintain access to new technology for Medicare or Medicaid that is similar to that of private sector insureds.

The view that, for the great bulk of the American population, higher health spending is worth it should be pressed more strongly. As part of this case, however, we should look seriously at (or for) the waste that many believe, based mainly on anecdote, is rampant in the medical care system. Either find the waste (and find a set of incentives to squeeze it out) or call the current outcome good—as good as it will get. While we may wish that improvement in the quantity and quality of life came more cheaply and easily, we will need to face the fact that, even at high real cost (with adequate protection for the uninsured), we do not want to reject what is still a bargain.

Index